Meditation

Meditation: The Ultimate Beginner's Guide for Meditation How to Relieve Stress, Depression, and Fear to Achieve Inner Peace, Fulfillment, and Lasting Happiness

Table of Contents

Introduction

Understanding Meditation

Why Should I Meditate?

How Will It Help Me?

It Comes In Many Forms

Types of Meditation

Focus Attention Meditation

Open Monitoring Meditation

Effortless Presence

Learning to Meditate

Types for Beginners

Preparing For Meditation

Step-by-Step Practice

Breathing Meditation

Mindfulness Meditation

Body Scan Meditation

Dealing With the Obstacles

Am I Doing It Right?

Squeezing Meditation Into Your Daily Life

Conclusion

Introduction

Have you ever thought about cleaning your mind? You know, taking it out and rinsing under water until you get rid of the clutter that overloads you? Have you ever wished you had the power to simply switch your brain off? Do you long for calmness?
No, we can not give our mind a shower, nor there is a switch that can stop it from overthinking so that we can put our focus solely on the things we do at given moments. But we can surely train our mind to do so.

Wait, before you put your kindles down, this isn't just a book that promotes the path of enlightenment and getting in touch with the spiritual. For you to instill stillness in your mind so that you become stress-free and relaxed, it doesn't matter if you are a religious person or a skeptic. This is not a book about Buddha. This is a book about you becoming aware and happy.

Meditation promotes stillness, awareness, and happiness. I will not lie to you and tell you that to achieve such a balanced state of mind is easy, because it is most definitely not. Just like every sportsperson needs a great trainer, you will need someone to guide you and show you how to practice this technique, as well. Fortunately, you have come to the right place. From explaining exactly what meditation is and what isn't, to teaching you how to train your mind and how to know if you are on the right track to becoming aware, while overcoming all of the obstacles that get in your way, this book will help you put the stress, fear and anxiety behind you. A person who meditates cannot be depressed or have mixed emotions. Those who meditate live in the present - calm and with sharp senses.

Let this book show you how to stop living on autopilot; let it help you find the peace within you that can bring the lasting happiness in your life.

© **Copyright 2016 by Lee Douglas - All rights reserved.**

This document is geared towards providing exact and reliable information in regards to the topic and issue covered. The publication is sold with the idea that the publisher is not required to render accounting, officially permitted, or otherwise, qualified services. If advice is necessary, legal or professional, a practiced individual in the profession should be ordered.

- From a Declaration of Principles which was accepted and approved equally by a Committee of the American Bar Association and a Committee of Publishers and Associations.

In no way is it legal to reproduce, duplicate, or transmit any part of this document by either electronic means or printed format. Recording of this publication is strictly prohibited, and any storage of this document is not allowed unless with written permission from the publisher. All rights reserved.

The information provided herein is stated to be truthful and consistent, in that any liability, regarding inattention or otherwise, by any usage or abuse of any policies, processes, or directions contained within is the solitary and utter responsibility of the recipient reader. Under no circumstances will any legal responsibility or blame be held against the publisher for any reparation, damages, or monetary loss due to the information herein, either directly or indirectly.

Respective authors own all copyrights not held by the publisher.

The information herein is offered for informational purposes solely and is universal as so. The presentation of the information is without contract or any guarantee assurance.

The trademarks that are used are without any consent, and the publication of the trademark is without permission or backing by the trademark owner. All trademarks and brands within this book are for clarifying purposes only and are the owned by the owners themselves, not affiliated with this document.

Chapter One – Understanding Meditation

There is a great deal of misconception revolving around meditation, but the greatest one of all is that people usually think that meditating is about making the mind go blank. If you are one of those people, let me just clear that up right now and tell you that it isn't true.

There is absolutely no way for you to press the power button and turn your mind off.

Meditation isn't about not thinking, but rather training your attention by focusing your mind towards the *presence*. But what exactly is meditation? The dictionary definition of the word meditation means deliberation, contemplation, thought or something to reflect upon. However, meditation isn't a thought. To you, meditation can be everything, or it can also be nothing. There isn't a single definition that can describe the meaning of meditation, but I will do my best to make you understand what this ancient discipline is all about.

Meditation is not a goal, nor something you get; it is a path you choose to be at peace and serenity. A discipline that can bring order to your mind, while getting rid of the scattered thoughts that distract you. It is about opening your eyes and seeing what you weren't able to see before. About sharpening your senses and breathing the life in. About being aware of where and who you are. Meditation is about becoming happy. In short, meditation is a discipline that makes you aware, fully present, clears your mind and relaxes you.

Another misunderstanding is that meditation means worshiping. Many believe that while meditating you get in touch with the spiritual.

That doesn't necessarily have to be true.

Meditation can mean a lot of things, depending on the reason you do it. Some people meditate to be able to concentrate, some do it to find peace and have a tranquil mind, while others may do it to surrender to the divine. It all depends on how you define meditation. Maybe this sounds somewhat confusing at this moment, but once you start receiving the benefits that meditation offers, you will then be able to dig deep within you, and find what meditation really means to you.

However you define it, meditation means a practice that settles the mind. This discipline has been practiced for thousands of years, and while it may have started in temples and among Asian monks (I will not go into details about the birth of meditation; that is a different topic for another time), the western cultures have been successfully experiencing the benefits of meditation for many years now.

Why Should I Meditate?

Whether it is your breath, your body, an object in front of you, or a single thought, meditation is about bringing the mind to its natural condition. To explain it even better, think of a cluttered room. The floor is piled up with junk, but on the other end of the room, there is an object you need. Now, to get there, you must first pass through the jumble. So you start grabbing and tossing things only to clear your way. Wouldn't it be much simpler if the room was clean? If you haven't guessed already, the room is a metaphor for your mind. Let's say you are working on an important work project, but you cannot seem to focus. You think of what your wife said that morning, think how you have to get to your daughter's play on time, the phone in the other office starts to distract you, and on top of everything, your gut starts rumbling to remind you that you haven't eaten yet. Now imagine being able to simply put every other thought and feeling aside, and focus only on the project you are working on. Meditation can help you do that. And no. To those of you who are thinking that I am talking about how you should bring out the cushion, cross your legs and start meditating during work hours so you can finish your project, I am not talking about that. Remember how I said that meditation is a practice that trains the mind? Once you train it to achieve focus, no one can take that away from you. It's just like riding a bike. Once you learn how to do it, that's it, you know. You don't have to go through the process of learning every time you wish to go for a ride. When you are trained to do so, you do it effortlessly.

But meditation goes way beyond simply clearing your mind and helping you to focus. It also helps you get in touch with the inner you. Some of you must be thinking 'here we go', but wait before making assumptions; you will see that it makes perfect sense. Answer me this, do you feel that your soul hasn't grown? We may look older than a couple of years ago, but if you do a little self-searching, you will see that the inner you hasn't aged a bit. You know how they say 'I look old, but I feel young'? The spirit doesn't grow or age. You learn new things, and maybe become more educated and know a lot more than you did a couple of years ago, but you still feel the same. The inner you is up for adventures, the inner you want to feel good, the one within you is the one that feels joy. Meditation helps you awaken your soul so that you can feel young constantly. And who would say no to that?

How Will It Help Me?

How many times have you said to yourself 'to finish that and I will finally be able to relax'?

There is always something. Our lives and daily routines are programmed to follow strict patterns, and each time we finish something, another responsibility pops out. You think after I settle this deal at work, then I can relax at last. How exactly do you relax? Do you take a week off and go on an exotic trip? Do you take two days to simply do nothing, put your feet up and watch your favorite show? Sure, that will knock down or should I say suppress the anxiety for a while, but what happens when your vacation is about to end? What happens when you're flooded with a million things that you have to take care of? Would you let the stress right back in?

Besides being a great stress-relieving tool, meditation can also help you with every aspect of your life, and that is something that has been scientifically proven. Still a skeptic? Read on to see how you can benefit from only a couple of minutes of meditating daily:

Meditation Knocks Depression Down.

Meditation is the best antidepressant drug. There are many ways in which this practice can decrease depression. The first one is that it boosts some brain chemicals like serotonin and norepinephrine, which are linked with depression. While taking a pill can also increase the levels of these chemicals, the effect is short-term (not to mention the possible side-effects that these kinds of medications carry), while meditation is long-lasting. There is a part of our brains that is called hippocampus, and it is known for disorientation (which depressed people are known for having) and memory loss. Studies have shown that people who meditate have an underdeveloped hippocampus, which is another indication how meditating can save you from this vexing disorder.

Meditation Relieves You From Stress and Anxiety. Meditation helps you concentrate, and I believe that is the biggest reason why it reduces anxiety and stress.

Anxious people are 'all over the place'. They are constantly chasing the tornado of spinning thoughts inside their heads. With meditation, the mind is focused. There are many studies which have proven this to be true. For example, one study performed by the University of Wisconsin Medison has shown that Vipassana meditation reduces the gray density in those areas in the brain that are associated with stress and anxiety.

Meditation Increases Your Pain Tolerance. The University of Montreal performed a study on 13 Zen masters and 13 people who didn't meditate. They exposed all of the participants to the same degree of painful heat and monitored their brain activity on an FMRI (functional magnetic resonance imaging) scanner. The Zen practitioners showed significantly less pain than the people who didn't practice meditation.

Speaking of pain, there are other studies which have shown how meditation can work much better than morphine.

Meditation Decreases the Risk of Heart Diseases. One research performed on a group of people who were at high-risk of having a heart attack, has come to some amazing results. The participants were asked to either take a Transcendental meditation class, or a class that promoted healthy diet and exercise. The researchers tracked their progress for five years. Those people who chose to take a meditation class did much better and reduced their risk of heart attack and strokes by an amazing 48%.

Meditation Decreases Blood Pressure. If you are one of those people who are at constant war with hypertension, know that choosing to meditate is probably your best weapon. One study performed on people with blood pressure has shown that after three months of meditating, over two-thirds of the participants reduced their blood pressure and dropped their need for medication.

Meditation Improves the Focus. Concentration, attention, and focus are probably the quickest-to-get benefits of meditation. If you thought that you should spend years of meditating to be able to increase your concentration, then you were so wrong. Since the focus is practically the main aim in meditation, know that if you do it the right way, you can achieve it after only a couple of days of meditating.

Meditation Reduces Addiction. Since meditation has such a significant effect over the area of self-control in the brain, it is understandable how it can reduce addiction and increase the self-control. For instance, there is one study that was performed on smokers who practiced mindfulness meditation and smokers who followed the freedom from smoking program (a program created by the American Lung Association), that has found out how those who meditate are much more likely to quit smoking than those who follow other programs that help people quit.

Meditation Makes You Happy. Researches show that only a couple of minutes of meditating every day can make you happier. According to these studies, meditation increases the brain signals in the left prefrontal cortex that is in charge of positive emotions, while it decreases those in the right prefrontal cortex that, which is responsible for negative emotions

Meditation Can Strengthen Your Relationship. Meditation may not have the power to affect the relationships you have with people directly, but many of the benefits you will receive while meditating can help you do just that. For starters, meditation improves empathy and compassion, which can boost your loving attitude for yourself, as well for other people, which will clearly change your point of view. For instance, if you used to get upset about small and unimportant things, meditation can help you see clearly, and they will not bother you anymore. Meditation can also increase acceptance and make you a better person.

Meditation Improves Your Sleep. One of the rewards that meditation gives its practitioners is a good night's sleep. If you meditate, you will not only improve your mood significantly in the long haul, but you will also be able to postpone the activation of the stress hormones before your bedtime, which will allow you to sleep like a baby. A study performed by the University of Utah has shown that mindfulness meditation promotes a good sleep.

But that is not all. The list of benefits you can reap off while meditating is pretty lengthy. The next are all scientifically proven benefits:

- Meditation strengthens your immune system

- It decreases inflammatory disorders

- It prevents asthma and rheumatoid arthritis

- Meditation reduces the risk of Alzheimer's

- It has an important impact on managing the respiratory rate and heart rate

- It slows down the aging process

- Meditation extends longevity

- It boosts creativity
- It improves the process of decision-making
- It reduces the symptoms of panic disorders
- It can help students to improve their grades
- Meditation supports weight-losing goals
- It increases tolerance
- Meditation improves social skills
- It improves skin resistance, and so much more.

The best part about meditating is that you can still enjoy its rewards even when you are not meditating. Remember the example from earlier about the work project? Meditation is long-lasting, and you can enjoy its benefits even when you are not practicing this discipline. Meditation makes changes in the brain's response to emotional stimuli, and that effect stays strong, even when one is not actively meditating.

It Comes In Many Forms

Many people believe that there is only one way to meditate and that meditation is one of a kind; that it has just been amended so that it can suit everyone's taste better. So that the

West can find beauty in it and stop thinking of meditation as something exotic. Crossed legs, closed eyes and 'empty' minds is how usually

people who don't meditate imagine meditation.

To those who don't understand this technique, meditation looks the same no matter how they call it. Those who think this, clearly haven't been rewarded with what meditation offers.

Depending on what you want to achieve, meditation can have many forms, and it can be done differently. However, they all share one thing in common – they all need the

practitioner to delve deeply into the depth of the mind, exploring self-awareness and consciousness. This exploring can be done from a different angle.

Types of Meditation

Meditation can be practiced in different forms. If you take a look at a group of people who are meditating, you would naturally think that they are doing the same thing, but that is very unlikely. Each type of meditation requires a different approach, and while on the outside it may look the same, the truth is, every meditation type is very unique, has a one of a kind procedure, and offers different results.

There are also those people who think that religion is what separates the meditation types from one another. They think that, whether you do it for the spiritual enlightenment and to get closer to the divine, or you are simply a nonbeliever who chose to meditate in order to regain the concentration and self-control, is the only thing that differentiates the individuals who meditate. Although, I cannot rule this one out completely, that is a wrong way of looking at meditation.

How you approach, where you put your focus, and what you allow to go through your mind while meditating, is what distinguishes one meditation technique from another, not whether you believe or not. There are religious and spiritual forms of meditating surely, but meditation has such a broad meaning, that if we make the difference based on religion, we will miss the true context.

Each way of meditating takes a different brain wave pattern which decides what the meditation will result in. That is why I say that you should choose the type of meditation based on what you want to accomplish by meditating.

Now, for you to gain a better understanding, I have divided the different types of meditation into three categories:

Focus Attention Meditation

I am sure you have already guessed that this type of meditation is for those who want to work on their focus and ability to concentrate. Focused attention meditation requires turning off the inner voice and cleansing the mind from the random thoughts, by shifting the focus to something else, whether we are talking about an object in front of you, a part of the body, a mantra, visualization, or something as simple as your breath. The point in this kind of meditation is to draw your attention to a single thing and get rid of the distracting thoughts or senses that may try to pull you back into the moment. Below you will find which meditation techniques fall under this category:

Some Forms of Zazen. Zazen or Zen meditation is a seated meditation with roots in the Chinese Zen Buddhism. Zazen can be practiced in two ways, depending on whether you want to focus your attention or to simply 'sit in the present'. At this moment, we will discuss the first one. Those who practice Zazen, use their breaths as the main focus on the exclusion of everything else that is going on around them. Zen practitioners say that Zazen is a very centering and calming way to bring order to our busy minds.

Loving Kindness Meditation. Loving-kindness or Metta meditation is another concentration technique, only here, the practitioner doesn't put his focus on the breath, but on his loving state of mind. That means that the focus of attention of the Metta meditation is the feeling of love, kindness, and warmth.

Chakra Meditation. Chakra meditation is a technique where the person who meditates focuses on one of the chakras (centers of energy) of the body. The practitioner focuses on one and tries to 'open' it, by feeling the

energy that flows through that area. Most of the chakra practitioners focus on the third eye (which is sort of like a sixth sense), which can provide the practitioner with a perception that is beyond what we can ordinarily see.

Mantra Meditation. To focus on a mantra means that the practitioner should recite a mantra over and over, silently in his mind, throughout the meditation process. To make it clear, Mantra is not an affirmation you say to yourself when you are sad or lonely, as many people think. The Mantra is simply a word that has no particular meaning, or it can even be a syllable. Some people think that the choice of the mantra is important and should have a 'vibration' that sticks, while others think that what the mantra will be is really not that relevant, as it is only something to put your focus on.

Sound Meditation. As the name indicates, sound meditation is a practice where the person who meditates puts his focus on sound. The sound you choose is really irrelevant. Whether you choose to play relaxing music on your smartphone, listen to the chirping of the birds, or sit on a beach and focus on the sound of the waves crashing down, the important thing is to put your attention on a single sound and disconnect from the thoughts in your mind.

Open Monitoring Meditation

Rather than putting your focus on a single thing and excluding everything else, open monitoring meditation involves monitoring every aspect of what we experience. To monitor openly means to observe everything that is going on around you. It means becoming aware of the present. The tricky part about this meditation is the fact that the practitioner shouldn't 'attach' to objects, sounds, feelings or

thoughts. The practitioner should observe and be aware of everything that is going on, but not to get himself into details because that means slipping from the meditation practice. When such a thing happens (it is normal for beginners to need time to train themselves), the practitioner returns to where he started. Open monitoring is not about wondering why or how something happens, but simply noting that it is there.

Since open monitoring allows people to focus on different things, it doesn't necessarily have

to be a silent meditation. You don't have to sit or close your eyes to be aware of the presence. You don't have to stop your daily activities to

practice this meditation; it can also be done while you do your normal activities. For instance, you can do it while playing guitar.

Focus on that. Focus on how your fingertips touch the strings, on the sound the guitar makes, on the way you feel while playing, etc. Here are meditation techniques that are open monitoring:

Mindfulness Meditation. We hear the word 'mindful' almost everywhere nowadays. It is

like it has become a buzzword that they stick it as a label on almost everything. But do people really know what it means to be mindful? To become mindful, one must have the ability to be present, aware and to observe things without judging them. That can be achieved through the practice of mindfulness meditation. Mindfulness meditation is concerned only with the present and the things that happen while you meditate. You still need to focus your attention, but unlike the focus

attention meditation, here, you don't focus on

particular things, but put on the present and all the things that happen then.

Vipassana Meditation. Vipassana means seeing things as they are. This ancient Indian technique helps the person who meditates to transform himself through the process of self-observation. Vipassana meditation helps the practitioner to gain a clear insight of the connection of his mind and body, while observing his thoughts and physical sensations carefully and slowly, one by one, moment by moment, without attaching to any.

Effortless Presence

The effortless presence is the state when the practitioner doesn't place the attention

anywhere, but simply sits steadily and silently, in peace. This is more of the desired outcome of the meditation than it is a type of meditation, really. This final stage is where the practitioner is well-trained and doesn't need a tool where he

will place the focus, but instead, he can effortlessly enjoy simply being. All of the quotes about meditation speak of this state.

The effortless presence or 'pure being' is the main purpose of meditation because once achieved it will reward the practitioner with ultimate relaxation, peace, and long-lasting happiness.

There are also some meditation techniques where the effortless presence is practiced from the beginning, and it is the only focus: some forms of Taoist meditation, Self-Inquiry meditation and some more advanced forms of Raja Yoga. However, one cannot simply start with the effortless presence unless he has some previous experience in meditation, therefore, I don't recommend you to jump-start this journey and start practicing such a challenging type because it will be extremely hard and you may end up disappointed.

'What type of meditation will suit me best?' Is the question that most beginners ask. However, the question you should really ask yourself is, 'What do I want to achieve from meditation?'. Perhaps, a person who is hard on others and wants to improve the relationships with other people may find loving-kindness meditation to be his best fit. But know that whatever type of meditation you choose, spiritual or secular, one thing is for sure. To truly benefit from this discipline, you need to start small and work your way up. Read on to see how to learn to meditate and work on your focus and discipline as a beginner.

Learning to Meditate

Have you ever taken a look at a group of toddlers playing in the park and thought how happy they were? Did you envy their carelessness at that moment? I bet you wished you could go back in time when there were no bills to pay, not a care in the world. Back to the time when your only responsibility was to show up for lunch, wash your hands, eat your veggies and go back to play. The time when your brain wasn't overburdened with too much

information. The time when all you had to do was sit and listen to your mother yelling about the mess she had come home into. The time when once she had made her point, you started plotting your next adventure. No kid spends time thinking about the past. Now, who doesn't

wish to live like that? But, what if I tell you that you can, in fact, learn how to feel careless again? What if I tell you that you can really learn how to stay in the present, not wasting your time worrying neither about the future, nor the things you should or shouldn't have

done? Learning these next meditation techniques for beginners will teach you how not to dwell on the past, but leave happily in the present.

Types for Beginners

Even as a beginner and with zero meditating experience, you can start practicing every type of meditation you want. Now, whether it will work or not, that depends solely on how strong your determination will be. That is why those who teach meditation strongly recommend that beginners start with simple techniques and learn to work on their focus and their ability to stay steady, patient and disciplined. Because,

as I said, meditation is not easy. It isn't

something you simply get over with. Meditation is not a performance, but a practice. And to practice means to spend time training.

I have picked some of the easiest beginner-level meditation techniques that will teach you how to slip into the gap between your distracting thoughts. Once you learn how to stay there, you will be able to concentrate effortlessly and take control over your thoughts, even when you are not actively practicing meditation:

Breathing Meditation. Some must be thinking 'how hard is it to breathe,' right? Well, of course, breathing on its own is easy, but putting your attention on the way you breath can be quite frustrating when different thoughts start interfering with your meditation. However, many agree that this is the simplest form of meditation, so it is probably a good idea for you to embark this journey with breathing meditation. It is a form of focus attention meditation and is recommended for beginners because the easiest way to meditate is to have something to put your focus on, and focusing on the way people exhale and inhale has proven to be more effective than shifting your attention to a sound or an object.

Simple Mindfulness Meditation. Do you know why this type of meditation is the most popular one? Since it was first introduced to the mainstream by the professor Jon Kabat-Zinn in 1979, mindfulness meditation has rapidly grown in popularity, simply because it is simple. To practice mindfulness meditation, you don't have to do anything else but

experience yourself, just as you are. You let go of all that burdens you, of all the negativity in your life, of the past, you let go of attachments, and most importantly, you let go of the

judgment. There shouldn't be any pressure.

You simply approach the practice with an open mind and a strong will to become truly happy in the present.

Body Scan Meditation. Although it is a part of the mindfulness meditation, I have decided to give the body scan meditation a special place on the list, since many beginners have succeeded in gaining awareness of the present, exactly by practicing this technique. By shifting your focus to all of your bodily parts, you will learn how to carefully observe, put your attention where you want, and also you will become able to shift your focus from one thing to another, without staying attached to what you were previously doing. This skill will especially come handy at work, right? Imagine being able to finish something and then shift and devote yourself to the next task, without letting the previous one distract you. This type of meditation can indeed boost your productivity.

Preparing For Meditation

Let's say a person wants to play tennis. To practice this sport, he will have to buy the necessary gear. From rackets and balls to tennis shoes and hats, that person must prepare himself for the actual training if he wants to learn how to play, right? Then, how is meditation any different? Meditation is also a practice, and it certainly requires a certain amount of preparation before you take a lotus posture and close your eyes. You cannot just dive into the depth of your thoughts out of the blue. People often neglect this fact and jump on the let's meditate train way too quickly. To truly enjoy the benefits of meditation, and avoid being just one of the many who tried and failed. Here are a couple of things you need to take care of first:

Exercise. Many meditation practitioners say that what helped them in the beginning was physical exercise. Your body has a significant influence on your mind, so it is only understandable how relieving the stress through exercise will jump-start your meditation and help you delve more deeply.

Try it out and see if this works for you. Of course, you should be careful not to overdo it, as in that case, the exercise will only have a negative impact on your meditation.

Take a Bath/Shower. Taking a bath or a shower before the meditation will get you in the mood for meditating since you will feel fresh and clean.

Choose Your Spot. Although the place where you will meditate is irrelevant, it is important that it makes you feel good. A dark and cluttered room is surely not a good spot for practicing. Try to make your meditation spot a beautiful, bright and clean place.

Get Comfortable. One of the most important parts of the process of meditating is that the practitioner feels comfortable. Always wear loose clothes that will not cause you discomfort during the practice. Also, if you tend to get cold, keep a blanket or a shawl nearby.

Ban the Distractions. Electronics and meditation simply don't work well together.

Make sure that your phone is on silent mode during meditation and avoid all other kinds of distractions. It is probably a good idea to let your family know of your meditating schedule so they will not interrupt.

Visualize. Knowing why you decided to meditate is important. Before each session, remind yourself of that. Try to visualize how you will feel once you start receiving the merits of meditation; once you go through life with a positive attitude, happy and unafraid. Visualizing the desired outcome is a great motivator.

Step-by-Step Practice

Before I start guiding you to the path of tranquility, self-awareness, and happiness, I want to tell you that it is okay to fail. At first, you may not even be able to take a decent posture, but don't let that discourage you.

Struggling to achieve clear focus is normal when you are a beginner; the important thing is to keep going, and once you succeed, you will never be lost in the maze of your thoughts ever again.

<u>Taking the Right Posture.</u> The posture is the spine of meditation. It is essential to adjust it the right way if you want to practice successfully. There is more than one way to meditate, and you can also do it sitting on your couch, lying in your bed, or even walking. However, to be able to meditate that way, you must first master *the lotus posture* (legs crossed), which I highly recommend for beginners. Here is how you do it:

Sit Down on The Floor. If your fancy meditation sitting down, the cushion can offer you a more comfortable seat, you can sit on it, however, many practitioners say how the cushions were kind of distracting in the beginning, and they preferred sitting on a flat floor.

Cross Your Legs. This one is really not a rocket science. Just cross your legs, but make sure you are comfortable.

Straighten Up. If you hunch down, you will never be able to learn how to do it right. Keeping a straight spine during meditation is the key to having calming results.

Relax Your Shoulders. The most common mistake that people make is that when they straighten the spine, they leave their shoulders tensed. Your shoulders should be relaxed and comfortable throughout the whole practice.

Placing the Hands. Place your hands right above your knees, to avoid being too stiff, as well as to keep your shoulders relaxed but not loose.

Your Head Should Be Comfortable. If you try to take a perfect lotus posture, you will notice that keeping your head comfortable is not as easy as it seems. The trick is to drop the chin slightly.

The Eyes. The important thing is not to keep your eyes wide open. You can meditate with loosened eyelids, but I prefer you to keep them closed, at least until you gain your focus.

Breathing Meditation

1. Get Comfortable. You can try rolling your head or shoulders if that does the trick for you, just as long you adjust your posture the right way afterward.

2. Breathe. It is recommended to do it through the nostrils and do keep your mouth closed. Don't think about it too much; there isn't a right or wrong way to

do it. Just observe your breath for about 2 minutes. Don't try to change the way you breathe, breathe normally.

3. Focus on the way the air enters and leaves your nostrils. Your focus should remain on this sensation, but you should also track the path that the breath makes in your body.

4. Imagine the breath flowing in and out of your body. Picture it entering the sinuses and lungs and the other way around. Know that distracting thoughts will most likely appear, it is normal. Simply, don't spend time dwelling on them and let them pass you. Return to your breath.

5. Feel how the space in your lungs expands each time you inhale.

6. Notice how it shrinks each time you exhale.

7. Feel how your chest rises and falls with each breath.

8. If you think it will be easier for you to breathe more deeply, then do so. Simply count to 4 while you inhale and count to 4 when you exhale. Just make sure that the length of the inhaling and exhaling remain the same. Focus on the lungs and chest as mentioned above.

9. Be sure not to control your breath.

10. If you start thinking about something else, slowly return your focus to the breathing sensation. Do this for as long as it takes until you settle on your breath.

Mindfulness Meditation

1. Start by taking a couple of deep breaths to relax and get you in the mood for meditating. Observe the breath as you

inhale and exhale. Feel the lungs expand and shrink.

2. Spend some time with your thoughts. Being mindful means being aware of the present, so whenever a stream of thoughts appears, spend time observing them closely. Imagine yourself floating or flying over them; so you can see each thought clearly. At this point, you shouldn't get into details, simply know they are there.

3. Now, it is time to become mindful of the thoughts. Focus on each thought separately. Why do you think that? Is it as a result of a previous event? Think of how it makes you feel. Do you want to feel that way?

4. Since at this point, you already know which thoughts you want to engage with, and which awaken sad feelings, it is time to dispute the unpleasant thoughts, so there is nothing but serenity inside of

you. This is somewhat challenging, and you might need a little bit more training to be able to release the bad thoughts, but know that only you have the power to do that, and if you try hard enough, you will succeed.

5. After you have released the thoughts that interfere with the meditation's goal, it is time to focus on your senses and be in the present. For instance, if you are meditating outside, focus on what you can hear. Focus on the sound that birds make. Focus on the way the fresh-cut grass smells, on the way that the wind tickles your skin, on the taste in your mind, etc.

6. Be aware that you will get distracted, whether by an unpleasant thought or a noise coming from the neighbor's house. When such a thing happens, simply return to the beginning and start with the deep breaths again.

7. Don't judge. Becoming mindful means gaining the ability to look at things nonjudgmentally. Meditating is challenging; don't judge yourself when you get lost in your thoughts. Start over and try again.

<u>Body Scan Meditation</u>

1. Just as the previous technique, start the body scan meditation with a couple of deep breaths.

2. Now, starting from top to bottom or the other way around, imagine your body divided into smaller parts. For instance, if you start with your feet, you will work your way up, and if you start with your head, you will then think, neck, shoulders and so on.

3. Focus on your head. Try to feel it. The heat, the vibration. Now divide it into

smaller parts: eyes, nose, mouth, ears. Try to 'feel' each part. Notice the sensation.

4. Move to your neck. Allow it to become 'soft' and relax.

5. Feel the shoulders. Are they tense or relaxed?

6. Move to the stomach area. Take a breath and let it soften as well. How does it feel?

7. Do this with each part of your body, breaking it into small pieces as you go. For instance, the arms should be divided into elbows, wrists, hands. The hands into fingers, knuckles, etc. Closely notice the function of each bodily part, as well as its relation to the other parts.

8. Try to feel the pressure, the heaviness, the pulsing. Try to relax.

9. When a distracting thought interrupts you, go back to the step number one.

<u>Ending The Practice.</u> There aren't any rules about the length of the meditation, but for the first couple of days, it is best to start with 5 minutes. You can start increasing the duration as you gain more confidence and become more comfortable.

When you are done, it is important to slowly return to the surroundings. Slowly open your eyes, and take a minute to move your shoulders or wiggle your toes before you stand up.

Dealing With the Obstacles

It is normal to get 'stuck' while meditating. It has happened even to the best. There is a way for you to overcome any obstacles that you may bump into on your way to attaining long-lasting equilibrium, but only if you want to. Before you go any further, it is important for you to find out whether you are determined enough. Determination is a must. Before you start purchasing candles and meditation cushions, make sure that you actually have what it takes to endure this challenging journey. Are you really strong-minded to receive the benefits of meditation? If so, then you will have no problem overcoming these next most common obstacles:

Irritation. Many fail because of the irritation. Whether it is an annoying noise that irritates them, or they are not comfortable enough, the point is, irritation can be an obstacle. *How to overcome it?* Simply by preparing yourself the right way, and ensuring you are comfortable before you start the session.

Doubt. Many people doubt their ability to achieve their ultimate goal through meditation and think that they don't have what it takes.

Thinking that those successful practitioners are better than you, can only crash your intentions before you even start meditating. *How to overcome it?* Spend some time examining yourself. Why wouldn't it work? Remind yourself of the qualities you possess and the things why you, too, can achieve what others can

Boredom. Some find sitting in one position for a certain period of time, to be boring. *How to overcome it?* If you feel bored, remind yourself of the reason you have started meditating in the first place. Spend some time visualizing yourself living relaxed and without fear. This may spark of your motivation if boredom pays you a visit.

Impatience. Waiting for 'something' to happen can be quite destructive. One of the reasons why not everyone succeeds in meditation is because of this obstacle. Everyone experiences meditation differently, and someone may need a little more time to achieve tranquility than others. *How to overcome it?* Only if you embark this journey prepared that it will take some time for you to taste the advantages of meditation, you can find your inner peace. Know that it will take some sacrifice.

Feeling Sleepy. It can happen for people to become sleepy during meditation, especially after long and busy day. Don't worry; this doesn't mean that you are doing something wrong, only that you really need a good night sleep. *How to overcome it?* Well, you don't, because this is not so much an obstacle, as it is a necessity. However, if it does bother you, you can try meditating first thing in the morning, or after an afternoon nap.

Am I Doing It Right?

Beginners get easily confused. It is normal to be unsure whether you are making progress and have started to receive what meditation has to offer, or whether you are still at that initial stage, learning how to attain a clear focus. 'Am I doing it right?' is something that new practitioners ask themselves. And while most teachers will tell you how meditation cannot be tracked nor planned, how you simply need to be and feel the moment, I disagree. On the contrary, I think that knowing exactly how you develop can have a significant impact on the goal you try to achieve. Otherwise, how will you know when it is time to move to a more advanced meditation technique?

Meditation is surely not something that can be easily monitored, and I agree with the gurus. But, the fact that you cannot put a measuring device and track the growth of the meditation directly doesn't mean that you cannot step back and observe the way in which this practice has changed you. That is how you will know whether you are doing it right or not.

Here are some tips:

- It is quite easy actually. Simply track how you feel after the sessions. Write it down. You can even create a table with different feelings, where you can simply put a check a couple of hours after the session, each day for 10 days. After ten days, you will see whether you have moved forward or not.

- Go on a trip for a couple of days and meditate intensively there. Once you get back and resume your daily activities, you can see if your mood has changed or not.

- If this doesn't help and you cannot seem to track your progress, then I suggest you stop meditating for 3-4 days. Stop practicing and observe your behavior closely. Do you notice something different? Has your mood changed? If so, then this is a clear indicator that you have been most certainly enjoying the benefits of the meditation.

Squeezing Meditation Into Your Daily Life

We live a pretty hectic life. Think about it. From the moment you wake up until you hug your pillow at night, your day is filled with busy schedules, stress, and worries. It seems like you are always in a rush, always hurrying somewhere. Who has time for meditation, right? Well, it doesn't have to be that way.

Maybe your eventful days don't allow you to reserve one hour to go to your favorite spot in the park and meditate, but that shouldn't be an excuse for you to stop practicing.

The best part about meditation is that it can be practiced anywhere and anytime. It isn't like practicing basketball; you don't need a hoop and backboard. All you need is your determination.

It may seem like an impossible thing to find time for meditation, but this chapter will convince you otherwise. So, no more excuses –

here is how you can squeeze this rewarding discipline into your daily life:

When You Wake Up. The trick is always to go for a morning meditation. If you think you don't have the time, then set the alarm to wake you up 10-20 minutes earlier. Ten minutes less sleep will not affect your beauty, but it will sure have a positive effect on your mood and behavior.

When You Have Time to Kill. Let's be honest, we are all so busy, but somehow we find the time to scroll through Facebook and Instagram. Instead of doing that, why not practice mindfulness? You don't have to adjust your posture and close your eyes, let's say in a restaurant, but you can indeed focus on the sensations you feel at that moment and recharge your batteries.

While Walking. Ever heard of walking meditation? It can be more challenging than seated meditation, but it is a wonderful time to practice and sharpen your senses and focus. Focus on the chattering, on the weather, on the faces of the people that pass you by. Anything around you can help you meditate.

Break It Down. Although of course, it is the most beneficial if you sit for 20 minutes, close your eyes and meditate, meditation can also be practiced during work hours. As a beginner, it is important to practice as much as you can, so it is recommended to seize every opportunity to focus. Try meditating on your lunch break. Reserve 5 minutes to simply clear your mind. You can also do it on bathroom breaks, or when you are alone in the office. 1-2 minutes a couple of times a day will indeed have an important effect on your progress.

Anchor It. Try to meditate for a few moments after each finished task. For instance, when you finish your lunch, you finish driving and park in your garage, after you go to the bathroom, etc. This way, every time you finish something, you will remind yourself that it is time for a couple of moments to quiet your mind. Before you know it, your focus will be sharp as a knife.

Conclusion

The road to enjoying the perks of meditation isn't sprinkled with petals. It is undeniable that it is a great challenge that requires patience, sacrifice, and strong will. That may sound intimidating, but it shouldn't. This book has the power to transform your mind completely and show you the beauty of the serenity if you allow it.

Only by practicing you will get to quiet your chattering mind. Now, go on, board this amazing journey to see how practice really makes perfect!

BEFORE YOU GO

If you liked this book, you might like these other books from Lee Douglas

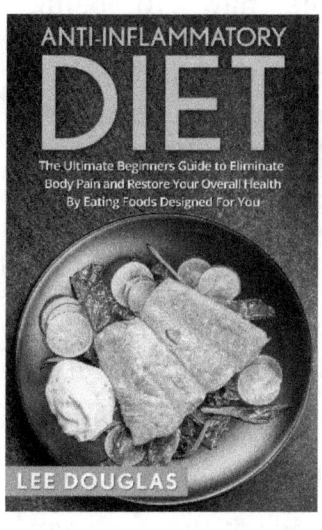 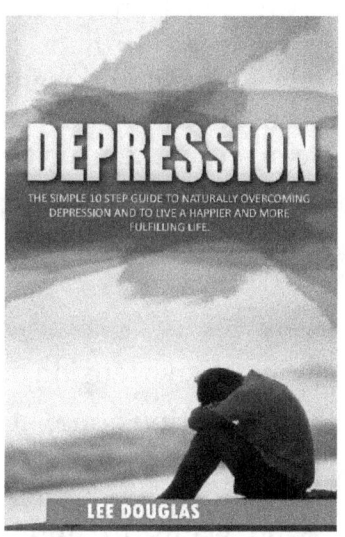

>>Check out more books by Lee Douglas<<

Chapter One – Understanding High Blood Pressure

You've just been to the doctor due to some disturbing symptoms, or maybe it was for something that you thought was simple, and know you've been diagnosed with high blood pressure. Hypertension, or high blood pressure, is not very uncommon in the United States anymore, and there seem to be one of two reactions that people have to being diagnosed with it. Some people are shocked they have it and want to find out whatever they can about the disease to determine how they can cure themselves of it, while others have heard of it so often they don't think of it as a threat to their health.

Well, hypertension is a threat to your health, and a serious one, at that. Since you're reading this book, I'm going to assume you're someone who wants to understand what they've been diagnosed with, and how they can overcome it.

So without further delay, let's get started with what hypertension is!

What is Blood Pressure?

Your blood pressure is the force at which your blood pushes against the walls of your arteries while your heart is pumping. When you have hypertension, this is when that force is too high. Your doctor will check your blood pressure with a gauge, electronic sensor, or a stethoscope. With this equipment, they will measure your systolic pressure, which is the blood pressure when your heart is beating and pumping blood, and your diastolic pressure, which is when your heart is at rest between beats. These two numbers make up your blood pressure reading, with your systolic pressure being first and your diastolic pressure being the second number.

Normal blood pressure for an adult is defined as being a systolic pressure that is below 120/80. It's normal for your blood pressure to change throughout your day, such as when you wake up when you're sleeping, and when you're nervous or excited about something. When you're active, it's normal for your blood pressure levels to rise, and when you stop being activity, your blood pressure ought to return to its normal rate.

Blood pressure will normally increase as you get older and if you gain weight. A newborn baby will have a low blood pressure number that's considered normal, while an older teen will have a number similar to an adult.

An abnormal blood pressure is someone who has a reading over 120/80.

While blood pressure increases seen in those who are prehypertension are less than those who are diagnosed with hypertension, prehypertension is able to progress into hypertension and should be taken seriously. Over time, a consistently high blood press will damage and weaken your blood vessels, which can lead to some serious complications.

There are two main types of hypertension. These are primary and secondary hypertension.

Primary hypertension is the most common form of hypertension. This form tends to develop over the years as you age. Secondary hypertension is caused by a separate medical condition or use of a medication. This type will usually resolve after the cause has been treated or removed.

What are the causes of high blood pressure?

Changes due to your genetics or your environment can cause hypertension, including changes in your salt balances and kidneys, your sympathetic nervous system, your renin-angiotensin-aldosterone system, and your blood vessel structure and its health.

Changes in your kidneys can cause hypertension. The kidneys tend to regulate your body's salt levels by retaining water and sodium while excreting potassium. Imbalances in your kidney function can expand your blood's volume, which can cause hypertension.

The renin-angiotensin-aldosterone system is what makes the aldosterone and angiotensin hormones. Aldosterone controls how your kidneys balance the fluids and salt levels, and angiotensin constricts your blood vessels. Increased aldosterone in your system or activity can change your kidney function, leading to hypertension due to high blood volumes.

Changes in your sympathetic nervous system can also cause hypertension. This system has imperative functions in regulating your blood pressure, including your actual blood pressure, heart rate, and your breathing rate. Researches are still investigating into whether or not imbalances in this system are the cause of hypertension.

In addition, changes in your actual blood vessel structure and function can also cause hypertension. Changes in both the small and large arteries can contribute to hypertension. The angiotensin pathway and your immune system can stiffen the small and large arteries, which will affect your blood pressure levels.

There can also be genetic causes of hypertension. Much of the knowledge about hypertension has been derived from genetic studies of the diseases. Hypertension tends to run in families. Years of research has identified a few genes and other mutations that are associated with the condition. However, these known genetic factors tend to account for only two to three percent of all cases of the condition. Emerging research suggests some DNA changes in the course of fetal development can also cause the growth of hypertension later on in your life.

An unhealthy lifestyle, such as a high amount of sodium intake, as well as sodium sensitivity, can cause hypertension. Also, drinking excessive amounts of alcohol and smoking are contributing factors. Lack of exercise that leads to obesity is also another factor that can contribute to hypertension, and some medications have been shown to be conducive to causing this illness.

Who is at a risk of developing high BP?

There are numerous different causes of hypertension, but there are some risk factors that you should be aware of.

First, age is the most common risk factor. As you age, your risk of developing hypertension increases greatly. Around sixty-five percent of Americans who are over the age of sixty have hypertension. However, the risk for this ailment is rising for children and teens due to the rise in the number of overweight children and teens.

Second, your ethnicity can be another contributing factor. Hypertension is more common in African Americans than in Hispanic American or Caucasian adults. Compared to these ethnic groups, African Americans tend to have hypertension earlier on in life, have a higher blood pressure number, and are less likely to achieve their goals for hypertension treatments.

Men are more likely than women to develop hypertension before the age of fifty-five. However, after the age of fifty-five, women are more likely than men to develop it if they have not already.

The most important factor is a family history of hypertension. If you have any close relatives, such as parents or grandparents, who have the disorder, then you are at a higher risk of developing hypertension. Genetics plays a large role in the development of this disease, so you should be checked out often by a doctor if you have a family history of it.

What are the side effects of hypertension?

While hypertension might not seem like the most frightening diagnosis at first, there are some serious side effects that should be considered.

First and foremost, aneurysms are a serious side effect of hypertension. This is when there is an abnormal bulge in the wall of one of your arteries. Aneurysms occur and grow for years without causing symptoms or signs until they finally rupture, grow large enough to press on a nearby body part, or block the blood flow. The symptoms and signs that develop will depend on the location of the aneurysms, but they are very life threatening.

Second, chronic kidney disease is another disease caused by hypertension and the two feed on one another. As the blood vessels in the kidneys narrow, hypertension becomes worse. This can eventually lead to kidney failure.

The next side effect is cognitive changes. Research has shown that, over time, hypertension can lead to cognitive changes. Symptoms and signs will include difficulty finding words, memory loss, and losing focus while you're having a conversation.

You can also experience damage to your eyes. This occurs because the blood vessels in the eyes will bleed or burst due to the pressure. The signs and symptoms include changes in vision and, eventually, blindness.

Of course, most people associate hypertension with heart attacks, which is absolutely true. When the flow of oxygenated blood to a section of your heart muscle is suddenly blocked and it doesn't get enough oxygen, you experience a heart attack. The most common symptoms are upper body discomfort, chest pain and discomfort, and shortness of breath.

Related to heart attacks is heart failure. When the heart is not able to pump enough blood to meet your body's demands, you go through heart failure. The symptoms of this include feeling tired, shortness of breath and trouble breathing, and swelling of your legs, ankles, feet, veins in your neck, and your abdomen.

Peripheral artery disease is a disease where plaque builds up in your leg arteries and affects the blood flow to your legs. When you have symptoms of this, the most common ones are cramping, pain, aching, numbness, heaviness of your feet, legs, and behind after you walk or climb stairs.

Finally, stroke is another side effect of untreated hypertension. When the flow of oxygenated blood to portions of your brain is blocked, stroke happens. The symptoms include an abrupt start of feebleness, paralysis of your legs, face, or arms, and trouble speaking or seeing.

What are the benefits of lowering high BP?

Of course, the main benefits of lowering your blood pressure is lowering your risk for developing all of the aforementioned ailments.

You'll be able to avoid heart complications. Hypertension puts a strain on the heart, which increases your risk of peripheral artery disease, angina, heart attack, coronary artery disease, and heart failure. Damaged arteries that result in hypertension collect plaque become hardened, and then narrow. Over time, the heart will become damaged and it will enlarge. The damage to your heart cannot be undone. Lowering your blood pressure to a normal level will prevent any future damage and help mitigate any previous damage by allowing your heart to work under the best conditions.

You will also avoid the risk of stroke. Hypertension puts a strain on the blood vessels throughout your entire body. When a blood vessel in your brain becomes blocked by a clot or bursts, a stroke occurs. Chronic hypertension is a risk factor for hemorrhage stroke, and the potential damage caused by hypertension contributes to ischemic stroke. Getting your hypertension under control can reduce your risk of developing a stroke, but it will not reduce the complications associated with a stroke.

You'll also improve your vision if you get your hypertension under control. Hypertension is known to put a strain on the eyes. The damage to your vision caused by hypertension will build up over time. Lowering your blood pressure to a normal level will reduce the strain that's put on your optic nerve, which is the nerve that is responsible for your ability to see. Uncontrolled hypertension can lead to hypertensive retinopathy, which is a disease that affects your eye's retina.

Lastly, you'll boost your kidney health. Your kidneys produce the hormone that helps regulate your blood pressure. Hypertension will damage your kidneys, and once they've been damaged, they will no longer help regulate your blood pressure. Lowering your blood pressure prevents this vicious cycle from occurring, and lowers your risk for total kidney failure.

Know how to measure your own blood pressure.

Knowing how to measure your own blood pressure at home can literally mean the difference between life and death. Depending on your condition, your doctor may instruct you to take your pulse regularly and determine what your blood pressure is. This will help you figure out if what you're experiencing is a true emergency or not.

So, before you check your blood pressure, there are a few things you need to do. First, you need to find a quiet space to do this. You'll need to listen for your heartbeat. Second, make sure you're comfortable and relaxed, and that you've recently emptied your bladder. Yes, your bladder being full can affect your reading. Third, you have to roll up the sleeve on your arm and remove any tight-sleeved clothing. Lastly, rest in a chair for five to ten minutes. Your arm needs to rest comfortably at your heart's level. Make sure that you're sitting with good posture, and you have your back against the chair and your legs uncrossed. Place your forearms on the table in front of you with the palm of your hand facing up.

To check your blood pressure, follow these steps.

1. Locate your pulse. You can do this by lightly pressing your index finger and your middle finger tightly to the inside center of your inner elbow. If you can't

find your pulse, then put the head of a stethoscope or an arm cuff in the same general region.

2. Secure the cuff. Thread your cuff end through the metal loop and slide it onto your arm, making sure the stethoscope is over the artery. The cuff can be marked with an arrow to show you the location of the stethoscope head. The lower edge of the cuff needs to be about an inch above the inner area of your elbow. Use the fabric fastener to make it snug, but don't make it too tight. Put the stethoscope in your ears and tilt the ear piece a bit forward to get a good sound.

3. Inflate and deflate your cuff.

   a. If you're using a manual one, hold the pressure gauge in your left hand and the bulb in your right hand. Close the airflow valve by turning the screw clockwise.

b. Inflate by squeezing the bulb with your right hand. You'll probably hear your pulse at this point.

c. Watch the gauge and keep inflating until it reaches thirty points above your expected systolic pressure. You shouldn't hear your pulses at this point.

d. Keep your eyes on the gauge and slowly release the pressure in the cuff by opening the airflow valve the opposite direction you used to close it. The gauge should fall just two to three points with every heartbeat.

e. Listen carefully for your first pulse beat. As soon as you hear that, note the reading on the gauge. This is your systolic pressure.

f. Continue to deflate the cuff. Listen until the sound disappears. As soon as you can't hear it any longer, note the reading on the gauge. That is your diastolic pressure.

    g. Let the cuff completely deflate.

4. Record your blood pressure. You should record the date, time, and the two numbers so that you can keep track of your blood pressure. Do this as often as your doctor recommends.

Finally, if you enjoyed this book, then I'd like to ask you for a favor, would you be kind enough to leave a review for this book on Amazon? It'd be greatly appreciated!

Thank you and good luck! ☺

www.ingramcontent.com/pod-product-compliance
Lightning Source LLC
Chambersburg PA
CBHW060409190526
45169CB00002B/821